Under the Sleeve

UNDER *the* SLEEVE

Find Help for Your Child Who Is Cutting

DR. STACEY WINTERS

NEW YORK

LONDON • NASHVILLE • MELBOURNE • VANCOUVER

Under the Sleeve

Find Help for Your Child Who is Cutting

Published in New York, New York, by Morgan James Publishing in partnership with Difference Press. Morgan James is a trademark of Morgan James, LLC. www.MorganJamesPublishing.com

ISBN 9781642798319 paperback
ISBN 9781642798326 eBook
ISBN 9781642798333 audio
Library of Congress Control Number: 2019950611

Cover Design: Megan Dillon megan@creativeninjadesigns.com

Interior Design: Chris Treccani www.3dogcreative.net

Editor: Todd Hunter

Book Coaching: The Author Incubator

Author Photo: R.J. Yuranek

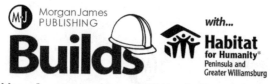

Morgan James is a proud partner of Habitat for Humanity Peninsula and Greater Williamsburg. Partners in building since 2006.

Get involved today! Visit
MorganJamesPublishing.com/giving-back

This book is dedicated to my mother and daughter who have loved me and supported my ideas for a lifetime.

Table of Contents

Introduction:	You Are Not Alone	ix
Chapter 1:	My Story	1
Chapter 2:	The Process	13
Chapter 3:	The Broken System	17
Chapter 4:	Cutting	33
Chapter 5:	A Child's Brain	43
Chapter 6:	Pathophysiology	57
Chapter 7:	Treatment	71
Chapter 8:	Obstacles	89
Chapter 9:	You Can Do This	97
End Notes		105
Suggested Reading		107
Acknowledgments		109
Thank You		111
About the Author		115

Introduction:

You Are Not Alone

This book was born out of the dream of reaching out to the many, many children out in the world who are suffering without the support they need. The key to overcoming any symptom associated with a mental health concern is that every child is different and has unique needs. The ability to discover those needs is rare and takes time. This required time is not supported by our current medical system. The cause of the mental illness crisis for our children is a monster subject debated and scapegoated incessantly. The underlying cause should be sought, finding it will help prevent. Meanwhile the issue at hand is that our children are suffering now, and we need to meet them where they are.

This mental health crisis is happening at this moment and is not constrained by location, economic status, race, or religion. It is absolute and is touching everyone, as it did for me and my child years ago and is now for millions of children who are suffering to the point they are cutting, suicidal, not engaging in life. This leads not only to possible suffering, self-injury, or the taking of a life. But when those moments of emergency are thwarted, what comes next? These children need help early and often. They need support from family, community, peers. They deserve to not be labeled or criticized. But how does a broken system overcome? Through education. Each individual must learn about mental health and its challenges. There should be no stigma only love and support and treatment. Each soul who can attempt to understand can then show another what it means to care and support a person in crisis. Individuals can amass into a tribe then into a force to change the world. We can change the system to support those with mental health concerns. If cared for in an appropriate manner and taught how to succeed at an early stage, these children can go forward into their lives equipped to succeed, not just survive. Everyone deserves to live a life filled with the idealism and a belief they can do whatever is in their hearts. Those with mental illness are no different. Families with children who have any type of mental illness deserve appropriate direction and support which can be done with education on the illnesses, education on the system, and the involvement of people who are dedicated and passionate to engage.

This mental health crisis, if not in your own home, is present in your family, circle of friends, or neighborhood. The majority of these crises are happening behind closed doors without outside support or awareness. It happened to Shelley, a working mom just like you and me.

Shelley's Story

Our lives had been as planned. I am an associate in a small law firm with a primary focus on family law working within an underserved community. It brings me such joy to be able to assist in alleviating crises for families in need. Charles, my husband, has succeeded beyond our greatest hopes after starting his architect firm. He built the vision I had in my head for our home. Not an easy feat, I must say. I have grandiose ideas and tend to skip the middle parts. But he succeeded beyond my wildest dreams.

We have three gorgeous children, Abby is 14, Michael is 12, and Maggie is 4. Maggie is a bundle of energy and a joy to all of us. She has bright yellow, ringlet hair, and is into everyone's things constantly. Michael is our serious young man. He, just like his father, loves numbers and solving problems. They designed and then built from all repurposed materials a three-room treehouse in the monster oak in the backyard. It is absolutely amazing. They make me so proud. Abby is a gifted artist. Any instrument she picks up, she can play a tune on by ear and she sings like an opera star. She also is scary intelligent. She never has to do much work or really even pay attention to get straight A's in school. Abby is the most loyal friend you will ever see. She supports those she cares about sometimes even to her detriment.

That old phrase "hindsight is 20/20" is true. Looking back, two years ago Abby became less engaged. Her playing the piano for fun decreased just a bit. Then she'd play only when we asked. She started going to bed earlier than the rest of the family or would spend the evening in the bath watching videos on her phone. I could hear her laughing at the videos and thought this was just what teenagers did. Her grades stayed good, still A's, but no longer high A's. Then 10 months ago Michael commented that he saw

Abby crying at bedtime. I walked into her room. She was bawling while curled up in a tight ball wearing her favorite pink flannel pajama pants. She could not tell me what was wrong. I asked about everything I could imagine – friends, a boy, schoolwork, teachers, physical pain. Nothing. She said she didn't know what was wrong. The next few weeks were back to normal, the new normal. She went to school, talked with friends on the phone, and halfway engaged in family activities. I had to ask her to join us at dinner and had to remind her to shower, take out the trash, pick up her room. When told to do her homework she said she didn't have any. It was then that I first noted her seeming sad. Nothing specific, just not quite as many smiles. Then I noticed no laughter when she spent time with her brother and sister. She stopped asking about my and her dad's work. I asked her if she was okay to which she repeatedly said, "Of course, mom. All is great."

Two weeks later, I saw lines of scabs on her left wrist. She had been wearing long sleeves every day for months I realized in that moment. After her two-hour bath that night, I went into her room. It felt so similar to the time months ago when I went in to comfort her. She was curled up on her bed in the same position although no tears this time. I asked her what had happened. She said she took a razor from her father's vanity and cut her arm. It was not the first time. She showed me areas on her thigh and her ankle. There were so many. Some mere scratches, some deep, some almost scars, and some appeared bright red as if they were about to bleed. My heart stopped. I wanted to scream and cry. But that would not help anyone. I asked what was wrong. How could she do this to herself. She said she didn't know. She was sad but there was no reason to be sad. I hugged her for hours. She cried quiet tears and fell asleep in my arms.

My child was hurting. It was my job as her mother to help. So I went to work. Where to start? It was 1 a.m., so Google was stop number one. I searched child cutting, self-harm, depression, how to help my child who is sad, treatment for pediatric depression.... There was information on crisis lines, lists of how to talk to your child, recommendations for therapy and to see your doctor. The websites all said to talk to your child and be loving and supportive. This we had been doing for years, really forever. It was how we chose to parent. That night I went over and over in my mind what had I done wrong that Abby would be so sad to cut herself. How could I have supported her more, recognized what was happening, prevented this? That next morning, I was on the phone with the pediatrician. We were in the office at her first appointment. She spoke with Abby after sending me to the waiting room. I was confused and hurting for my little girl. Dr. Charity referred Abby to counseling, spoke with us both about distraction if she felt like cutting and gave us a laminated bright green sheet with crisis numbers to call if she felt suicidal. I felt empowered. We had a plan.

The recommended counselor was not taking new patients. I called the pediatric office. Another referral was made. Two weeks later, we met Abby's counselor. She was about my age, dressed in a suit and in a crisp manner kicked me out at the onset. I was allowed back in at the end to ask questions. Abby just sat in the chair and looked at the floor. As soon as we were back in the car she started crying and said she hated that lady and did not see how that would help. Subsequent months of jumping through hoops with the insurance and trying different therapists did nothing. Abby did not feel comfortable talking to anyone. We tried all the online coping recommendations. We returned to Dr. Charity multiple times who eventually said Abby should probably be started on medication, but she did not feel comfortable treating pediatric depression. We were referred again. Abby just got worse. She cried almost every day, she stopped playing music and singing, she refused to eat healthy foods, she slept most of the day but not at night, she spent all her time on her phone – doing I do not know what. When I would get her up for school she would start crying and saying she could not go. She was nauseous and her stomach hurt. She would cry so hard she could not breathe.

My child is suffering. I do not know what to do to get her help. Who do I talk to? How do I wade through the medical system to find a person who knows what to do to treat Abby? How do I know what they are doing is right? Can she be helped? Will this last forever? Is this my fault? Will my heart survive?

Chapter 1:

My Story

Shelley's story is one I have heard over and over again in my practice from parents in every walk of life across the US. Her story is an accurate reflection of my and my daughter's saga. My journey to arriving here, sharing my story with you started long ago. This book incorporates what I have learned over 20 years in pediatrics about children suffering with mental health issues combined with my personal experiences seeking any possible relief for my child who has suffered with anxiety, depression, and cutting.

I was the epitome of a child growing up with a plan. My family was completely supportive and encouraged me along the way. From age four, I knew I was going to be a doctor and wanted to help others. Blind ambition with a utopian ideology backed by the ideal that all can be accomplished with enough desire and work was my driving force. This mindset got me to medical school, through residency, and into a thriving private practice. I purchased an independent pediatric practice near where I grew up in Oklahoma City. Yes, that was a thing back then. Twenty years ago, there were some children with depression and cutting. It was rare but present. Even then, I did not feel as pediatricians we were trained well enough in medical school and residency to provide the effective support needed for children with these concerns. I wanted to be able to treat them better. I sought to educate myself farther through research, reading, and attending as many continuing medical education courses on mental health treatment as possible. Life evolved as did my education, experiences, and expertise.

Over time, the practice of medicine changed. It was becoming impossible to stay afloat as an independent doctor practicing on her own. Many of my friends were giving up private practice to become employed by the big conglomerate systems taking over medicine. This seemed liked a good opportunity for my family to move and experience life outside of Oklahoma. The subsequent moves allowed me to experience many types of practices and medical delivery systems. I was employed by a community hospital in a small town where gangs, marijuana use, and depression were rampant. My family and I then moved from that tiny town in Washington state to a larger community where I practiced as a pediatric hospitalist for a regional medical center. This was a time where I felt even more drawn to pediatric mental health. It was there I saw many of the more acute tragedies which can accompany young children suffering with mental health concerns and experienced firsthand how they were not getting the help they needed.

As pediatric hospitalists, we admitted all children to the pediatric floor who had attempted suicide or were too intoxicated with alcohol or drugs to go home. We also cared for the children with significant mental health concerns who could not go home. These kids had to wait for possible placement in an appropriate mental health institution for further evaluation and treatment. One such admission to the floor was a seven-year-old girl. She was adopted and the parents did not know her complete medical history other than she was exposed to alcohol and drugs during the pregnancy and she was taken from her biological mother at eight months of age. She was in the foster system for a little over two years and then adopted by them at age three. Her behaviors had been challenging from the start. She would cry when hugged and refused most foods other than milk and chicken nuggets. Over time she seemed to adjust and become more comfortable with touch and affection. Her diet improved. She loved all foods and ate most fruits and vegetables. At the age of six, she started throwing extreme fits at bedtime. It would take them hours to get her to sleep. She would scream, cry, kick, and hit. She broke furniture and caused some bruising to her adopted father. They took her to their pediatrician who referred them to counseling. The counseling had no effect on her behaviors which continued to escalate.

She started self-harming just before her seventh birthday. Her parents discovered the cuts only because she did not think to get rid of the clothing which had been bled on prior to it being laundered. They asked her why she would cut herself and she answered that she did not know – then said she wanted to know what it would feel like. She used a kitchen knife. She was admitted to a short-term pediatric mental health facility at that time. She was there for five days and sent home. Her behavior was too much for them to handle. The facility did not feel it was safe for her to remain in their care. Over the next few months, this small girl physically attacked her adopted mother and caused a black eye, she threatened her father with a knife, threatened suicide, and cut again. They brought her back to the ER at my hospital desperate for help. She was placed on our service and stayed there. We requested a psychiatrist from the area to come see her on our floor as a consult to provide needed expert opinion. Her behaviors were more than we as pediatric hospitalists were trained to diagnose and treat appropriately. He recommended she be placed inpatient in a suitable mental health facility where she could be observed over time so that an accurate diagnosis could be made along with establishing an appropriate and affective treatment regimen. The social workers worked for weeks to try to find a place for her without success. There were no open beds or the facilities would not accept her due to her aggressive behaviors. She and her parents were on our floor for 13 days. We ended up having to send her home with community supports. She was not served in any way. To this day I do not know what happened to her or her family. I hope they got the help she needed to be treated for her illness.

It was during this time that my brilliant, sensitive daughter who always had difficulties with transitions developed depression and anxiety resulting in self-harm. Her father and I had divorced two years prior, then a traumatic event occurred in her life. I, to this day, believe this was the trigger for all that followed. She and I faced turmoil after turmoil. We did not have support from anyone other than my amazing mother who lived 1800 miles away. I am a physician. I treat depression and anxiety in my practice. How could this have been the impossible, painful task it was? At the onset, she vomited every morning for days. Once that was under control, she could not go to school. She was so sad and anxious she could not engage in life. She developed physical symptoms of severe headaches. I was going down the medical path of brain cancer or meningitis – but in the end, it was all due to anxiety. She started to cut and expressed suicidal ideation many times. I was one of the lucky mothers – she did not ever attempt suicide.

The fear and powerlessness were paralyzing. We could not find a physician who felt comfortable treating her with medications. I made her go to counselor after counselor. It is what I knew to do. But, she did not like the counselors – any of them. The counselors would ask me first what was happening with her. I would tell the story. Even when asked she would not share her thoughts or her perception of the history which brought us there. She would not talk. And talking is what counseling is all about....

My daughter felt the counselors we tried looked down on her, judged her, and treated her as if she was a small child. The connection needed to get through to her was just not there. She continued to go because I insisted even though she did not want to and felt it was not helping her in any way. She was not in a place where talk therapy could work for her due to her age, her biases and her brain chemistry not being balanced at the time. Our pediatric mental health system mandated counseling is what you do first, then if that fails you go on to the next available treatment option which typically is medicines. These counseling visits were only partially covered by insurance and were costing a fortune. She would go and sit there.

We could not find a physician who felt comfortable treating her with medications. Finally, a physician friend of a coworker of mine saw her and started her on an SSRI (specific serotonin reuptake inhibitor medication) to help with the depression component. The subsequent medication changes made over time were not because the doctor was confident in prescribing a course of treatment, but at my suggestion. As a mom, I should not have had to become involved in the care of my child with depression and anxiety. Her treatment should not have been based upon my medical knowledge.

She and I moved after a period of time, a change in setting I hoped would help. Fairly soon after the move she developed suicidal ideation once again. Nothing I said got through, I panicked, and called to set her up a visit with a PhD psychologist as an emergency visit. She saw the only one who had been suggested to me (there were three) who would work her in the following day – not schedule one month out. We had not previously been to a visit with a PhD. I was optimistic that the different type and extended length of training this particular doctor had would be a better fit for my daughter. Maybe this person would have the skill to reach her. My daughter went to the appointment and was angry after – the visit did nothing for her suicidal ideation. All the doctor of psychology did was an intake to get her background first from me then from her. Nothing was taught to her about how to distract herself to not go through with a suicide attempt. My daughter came out of that appointment infuriated. But, that in and of itself seemed to help decrease the deep depression and suicidal ideation. Needless to say, we did not go back.

I tried to teach her coping skills, meditation, every trick I knew and she would not listen to me. But, of course, I am mom, why would she. As she was placed on an additional medication that I recommended to her pediatrician, life went on – she got a bit better. After four years, we finally found a psychiatrist who was a fit for her. It took extensive searching and phone calls to find a physician who was taking new pediatric patients. It ended up being luck. I had been given a recommendation for a specific doctor. I contacted the office and was told she was full and not accepting new patients. That office gave me the name of another adolescent psychiatrist who might be open and taking new patients into the practice. I called and she was able to see my daughter the following week. The first visit was a bit rough. My daughter had been to so many practitioners she did not believe anyone would see or hear her much less be able to help. I made her go to the next scheduled visit. They made a connection on that second appointment and my daughter still goes to her for continued treatment. My daughter has evolved into a young adult who succeeds in what she puts her mind to and is evaluating where to take her life next. She still struggles on occasion with sadness and anxiety. I have to wonder what her youth could have been if we had the tools we now have in place when her problems first started. Of course, there is no way of knowing.

My approach to treating mental illness in children is built on the additional medical training I sought out over the course of my career, the struggles with finding help for my child, and my work experiences over time. I have had the pleasure of working in private pediatric practice, as a pediatric hospitalist, in primary care in underserved communities and in affluent areas of a big city, in child abuse, and as a pediatrician treating mental health issues full time. Over time and the varied organizations/locations it was clear. Our world is not equipped to help our children with mental health concerns. I currently work 60 to 80 hours per week seeing many children. I know I touch lives daily and am making a difference for many. I can only reach the few that come through my door and connect with me.

Seeing the children I have treated walking into the clinic smiling and laughing is a reward beyond measure. I have been able to reach many and help them stop self-injurious behaviors. I would love to be able to help find a way to reach those children before they act and prevent them falling into a place where self-harm is the answer. My job is to educate and direct so these kids can find care and develop the skills to be in charge of their own minds and emotions.

Chapter 2:

The Process

The only way to make effective decisions in life is to have as much of the available information as possible. As a parent, discovering that your child is suffering, your educated decision-making is the path to the healing your child requires.

Chapter Three will detail the broken pediatric mental health care system and how, through knowledge, you can navigate the system to find providers who fit your and your child's needs. There are many steps in obtaining appropriate mental healthcare and the options are often limited. There are roadblocks which would be hard to imagine. The system itself is not equipped to provide needed care. There are time limits on visits, not enough providers, providers who are unwilling to care for kids with mental health crises, providers who think they can but do not have the education or experience to do so. The pediatric psychiatric institutions themselves are too full, do not have enough staff, or cannot handle the situation. Families are often left to fend for themselves when placement cannot be found. The subspecialty needs for these kids are rarely met. There are just too few pediatric psychiatrists.

In Chapter Four, I will discuss the many possible reasons kids will begin cutting. When faced with an episode of cutting or discovering it has been happening for an extended period of time, it is best to understand what cutting really is. You will most likely never accept it but being able to communicate effectively with your child requires education about the process and the understanding that there is no blame to be placed on a parent or a child.

In Chapter Five you will learn about the process of development for a child's brain and how that affects their perception of emotions and therefore their behaviors. The needed education is not just on the action of cutting but also about the brain chemistry and development which accompanies or rather precedes the act. The brain of a child develops emotional maturity very slowly. Children do not understand themselves what is occurring with their emotions and feelings.

In Chapter Six the pathophysiology of pediatric mental health is discussed. You will learn that cutting is a symptom. The pathophysiology of depression and anxiety will be explained. These are not the only underlying conditions which can contribute to cutting and they rarely stand alone.

In Chapter Seven you will learn about treatment options and recommended therapies. Treatment for cutting is not directed specifically at the cutting. The underlying mental health process must be identified. To treat, an accurate diagnosis is a must. The treatment is based upon what is happening in the child's life and brain. The chemistry of the brain must be supported in order for other therapeutic interventions to have affect.

In Chapter Eight the obstacles you will face in obtaining appropriate effective mental health care for your child who is cutting are discussed. The village concept of treatment is one I embrace. Every family and child are unique. Their needs are unique. It takes different approaches to reach the needs of an individual. Your child deserves a physician who is versed in pediatric mental health diagnoses and treatment. This physician also needs to be working in a practice where they are afforded the time needed to establish rapport and gather all essential information to determine the proper diagnosis. Then a counselor or therapist who has a connection with the child is a part of treatment. Many children respond well to mindfulness techniques, so you will need a person who can teach those techniques and follow up on that learning. The family must continually seek education in order to participate in care and support the person who is hurting. The friends of the family and extended family need to be apprised if there are sensitivities and how best to interact or support the process. At times, the teachers and counselors in school will become involved. School participation can suffer and your child needs support by the school to stay in good standing. This is the old-world village where people come together in support of one in need. This is the time for such an approach.

Chapter 3:

The Broken System

There is a specific moment when a parent recognizes their child needs help for a mental illness concern. That moment can be the discovery of hundreds of red lines on her arm, under the sleeve of her favorite sweatshirt. It could be realizing she has not slept in two days or that she cannot go to school because she is crying to the point of losing her breath nearly every morning. It could be as drastic as a suicide attempt. No matter what the event or when the realization strikes, it is an absolute crisis. The fear and lack of power for a parent is beyond measure.

The absolute first thought parents have in this situation is that they need to get help. So many parents seek this help support by talking to family and friends. Some cannot reach out to these groups due to the stigma often associated with mental health concerns. The negative connotations are much more significant in certain cultures. Then you get the advice from Grace, your great aunt, who says this will pass just leave her alone. Your best friend says to keep her home and rub oils on her feet. Dad says make her go to school, she just needs discipline. Needing more than advice, you call the person who should logically be able to help – your pediatrician.

The Board-Certified General Pediatrician

To be licensed as a pediatrician and practice in the United States a person must complete a four-year bachelor's degree from a university or college, and four years of medical school. They then are trained in a pediatric residency for a minimum of three years. The residencies vary as to how much mental health diagnosis and treatment exposure is attained. It also varies based upon an individual's interest. Some doctors are not comfortable with treating mental health. Your pediatrician also may or may not be board-certified. Board certification is earned through testing then is maintained over time by meeting continued educational criteria set forth by the pediatric specialty board.

The pediatric office of today is not designed to manage or support mental health concerns much less a crisis. The appointment schedule is not managed by the doctors but by staff who typically do not have medical backgrounds. They often do not have the knowledge base to recognize an emergency nor the support structure to pass it on to the appropriate person if they do. The schedules are packed as full as possible for the highest possible number of visits. Most doctors are now employed by corporations and have no say in how the clinic is run or how their schedule is managed. Pediatricians who run their own clinic, who have complete control over their time, are for the most part a thing of the past.

The visits are commonly limited to 10 -15 minutes for acute complaints and up to 30 minutes for well child checks. Some offices will allow additional time for certain conditions such as mental health concerns, but only if there is a space or gap in the schedule. The additional piece, as you know, is that when you call for an urgent appointment you may be put with any provider who is available. You most likely will not be able to see your pediatrician because of the full schedule. So, you are in crisis over something scary and personal. You and your child now have to divulge intimate details to a person you may not know and you do not know their qualifications or experience with mental health.

A first time visit for a mental health concern in a child can take up to two hours if done properly. This time is needed to gain the trust of the child and gather all the information needed to determine the proper diagnosis. The first diagnosis may not be complete or could be designated as "to be determined" due to needing more time with the child and family to understand the full situation. We have a diagnosis we use of "behavior concern" for that purpose. If you try to cram into the typical ten-minute sick visit the required information gathering about how, when, and why a child is cutting, you will fail – not only in your diagnosis but in ultimate success. When you call in requesting an urgent visit for concerns of cutting, what typically happens is a ten-minute appointment is scheduled with whomever has an open slot. The provider you see does the very best job they can in that time frame and a referral is made. The referral can be to a counselor, another pediatrician, a specialist, or to the Emergency Department.

It is important to know what training the person who is evaluating your child has both overall and specifically in mental health.

Developmental Pediatrician

This is a subspecialty of pediatrics. A developmental pediatrician goes through training as a general pediatrician does. They then participate in another three years of additional training after the three-year general pediatric residency called a fellowship which centers on child development and behavior. They primarily focus on assessment, research, and treatment. An assessment with a developmental pediatrician is often multidisciplinary and will include evaluations with occupational therapists, speech therapists, and counselors. These evaluations tend to take a very long time to schedule, some of my patients have waited up to a year. Once the evaluation is set, the appointment can take one to two days consisting primarily of different types of testing. The results can be extremely helpful in treatment of some children.

Psychiatrist

Psychiatrists attend the same four years of medical school then start a residency in psychiatry. There are different pathways for psychiatrists. They can complete a three- to four-year residency in general psychiatry – all ages. An option exists where a three-year general residency is completed followed by a two-year fellowship specializing in pediatrics/adolescence, geriatrics, research, psychotherapy, etc. There is also a pathway where a pediatrician who completed a pediatric residency can attend a three-year pediatric psychiatry fellowship.

General or Family Practice Doctors

Family practice doctors follow the same undergraduate and medical school requirements as pediatricians. The family medicine residency is also a minimum of three years after graduating medical school. Their residency covers medicine from birth to death. They typically get three months or so of specific, designated pediatric training in the three-year program.

Physician's Assistant

A PA or physician's assistant completes four years of college then attends a two-year program similar to the first two years of medical school. Most states do not allow PAs to practice independently requiring a physician to review charts and oversee patients. They do not get residency type training but rather train under physicians in their field of choice.

Nurse Practitioner

The nurse practitioner profession was originally designed for RNs who had years of clinical experience to go back to school and then provide medical care at a level between nursing and physicians. This field has evolved greatly in the last decade. A bachelor's in nursing or other field is now the requirement to be admitted to a nurse practitioner program. There is no longer a requirement for clinical or work experience prior to matriculation. There are two-year and four-year programs. Those who complete the four-year program are designated as doctors of nursing. There are family nurse practitioners, pediatric nurse practitioners, psychiatric nurse practitioners, and other designations as well. The psychiatric nurse practitioners are trained in psychiatric medications and counseling practices.

Psychologist

A psychologist (PhD) completes a four-year undergraduate program and then a four- to seven-year doctorate. There are more than 30 subspecialties within the field. They tend to focus on research, theory, history or clinical practice. You will find PhD psychologists working in schools, governments, public or private corporations, and clinical practice. A behavior evaluation by a PhD can take one to two days of examinations and testing or can be an hour-long office visit. This type of evaluation can be extremely helpful in diagnosis and treatment but is not necessary for many children.

Counselor

A counselor is a person who provides talk or play therapy. Counselors can be trained in multiple approaches to therapy. Some are specific to children or appropriate to specific diagnoses. Their role in treatment can be extremely valuable. They complete a four-year undergraduate degree then a two-year master's program. The master's degree can be in counseling, social work or another related field of study. To become licensed and practice as an independent counselor they then complete 3,000 supervised clinical hours. Each counselor can tailor their training to the population or work environment which interests them. Counselors specialize in – family, individual, groups, substance abuse, psychoanalysis, learning disabilities, school, trauma, and more.

Crisis Lines

The crisis lines are now in place around the world. The purpose is to have a person to reach out to at any time day or night if there is a crisis. They were primarily founded for suicide prevention. These lines are manned by people who have had varied experiences and education. Some are volunteers, some full-time employees. All receive training on how to speak with a person in crisis. These centers also are engaged in the community. They will be able to provide resources and recommendations.

It is important as a parent that you have the knowledge about how the professionals who may be treating your child are trained. It is not that one type of provider is better than another. Their capabilities are determined by the experiences they have had in their career and education. Some will have further training in a field. Some have exposures to a certain population and therefore have much greater knowledge in that area. This is very important in pediatric mental health. Each professional is as unique as your child. It is your right and responsibility to ask about experience and competence. Most providers will be happy to know you are seeking the best care for your child. If they are offended by the questions, then they are most likely not a good fit for your family/child. You can ask the front staff scheduling the appointment if the provider sees pediatric mental health patients. If they do, how often? You can ask the provider about their experience in pediatric mental health. Have they seen the behaviors your child is now exhibiting? Have they treated this before? How? Are they comfortable with treating this type of behavior?

Choosing the person who will be working with your child through a crisis can be a significant challenge. Finding the person who has the training and the experience is a start, but then you must also have a personality match. Trust is paramount. A child needs to be comfortable opening up but also listening and following recommendations. Children and teenagers can tell in an instant if the person they are talking to is a fit. It is about the feeling and how the kids are addressed. Each child is different, and it may take them meeting different doctors, providers or counselors before deciding with whom they are most comfortable. This treatment is not for an ear infection where any person can look into the canal, see a red, bulging ear drum, and prescribe an antibiotic if indicated. Treatment is based upon correct diagnosis then time together, sometimes over years to find success.

Sometimes the extent and urgency of what is happening in the moment determines who and what level of care you seek for the issue. If you have discovered deep cuts or your child states they no longer want to live, it is time to seek emergency medical attention which cannot be provided at your pediatrician's office. Do not try to go to an urgent care clinic. They are not equipped and do not wish to treat mental health concerns in children. The emergency department is the only option available. I recommend if the need arises to go to a children's hospital. They will be better at complete assessment, communications with your child, and hopefully have better access to follow-up care than the adult varieties. Emergency departments are exactly what it sounds. They are trained to stabilize, treat the presenting problem as indicated then admit their patient to the hospital for continued care, or send them home with follow-up. The follow-up provider then has the responsibility for long-term diagnosis and treatment.

One of the greatest issues in pediatric mental health care (adults face this as well) is a gap in the system based upon acuity. If you go into the emergency department and your child has attempted suicide, he or she will be admitted to the hospital. After admission, it will be determined whether a higher level of care is needed in a psychiatric facility or not. If admission for psychiatric care is needed, then an appropriate facility must be found and then they will need to have room available. Another child who was admitted to my inpatient pediatric service at the regional medical center in Washington state was a 14-year-old girl. She had overdosed on Tylenol. The treatment for a Tylenol overdose takes two to three full days of medication given by IV. Being stuck in the hospital, over time she shared more with me about her life and situation. She was in advanced classes as a freshman in high school and felt a great deal of pressure to succeed. She was also very involved in music and drama. The opening of Little Shop of Horrors where she had the lead was happening in two months. The third day I saw her, she shared that she had been cutting and showed me her wounds. They were on her left forearm, right thigh, and the inside of both ankles. Most were superficial and appeared as thin red lines. There were a few which had scabbed over and would leave a scar. It took significant time and long conversations between her and me to convince her to tell her parents about the cutting. They reacted as you would have expected. They asked her why. Hearing about this long-standing self-injurious behavior on top of the girl's suicide attempt, they felt defeated. This patient, her parents, the social worker, and I, all felt she would benefit from a short stay in a lower level psychiatric facility for kids. Once she was medically cleared from the Tylenol overdose, she still felt intense depression, and was able to articulate that she still felt suicidal. She was at significant risk for a second attempt. She was kept on the pediatric floor for another week. As was the case with my younger child, there were no beds available. At the end of the week, she was sent home with her parents with a safety plan in place and instructions to seek out counseling. The "safety plan" is a good tool and is made up of a discussion held between you as the parent and a counselor or social worker about how to make sure the home is safe for your child. Typically, the safety plan details that all knives/sharp objects are secured, if there are guns, establish the proper and safe way to store them so there is no access, and how to lock up all medicines, again so there is no access. I worry the pressure this can put onto parents as the only responsible parties who are to protect their child in a crisis situation. I would like to see much better support in every aspect of hospital discharge following an admission for a mental health concern.

If you enter the emergency department with cutting or suicidal ideation, the gap in care compared to a hospitalization is evident in the style of treatment. It is not that they do not care. It's that the system does not allow the needed time and space. They will treat what is urgent at that moment, such as suturing wounds, or administering charcoal for an ingestion of drugs. If an inpatient stay is not warranted or indicated, a social worker will be called. They will arrive as soon as they can, which could be many hours. They talk with you about your home and establish a safety plan. They will also help set up follow-up – typically with your pediatrician.

The better you know the system, the better prepared you are to find the resources needed to get appropriate care, diagnoses, and treatment for your child. Ask questions. State your needs. If you do not feel your provider is the person that fits with you and your child, ask for a referral to someone else. Keep calling. No system is perfect. A referral may have been misplaced or not received. It is okay to self-refer. If you find a provider or counselor you think is a perfect fit, call, request an appointment. If you are told you need a referral, call your PCP (primary care provider), and request one. If they say no, then make an appointment with the PCP and get one. Insurance can also sometimes be a source of information on available options to investigate.

A perfect scenario would be for all the disciplines to bring together their knowledge and work in a cohesive manner to help our kids.

The scenario I see occurring more now is that there are not enough providers who treat mental health in children due to more instances and need for pediatric mental health care. But also due to an insufficient number of trained providers. This applies to pediatric psychiatrists, pediatricians trained in mental health, psychologists, psychiatric nurse practitioners, and counselors. A recent patient of mine came to me in full crisis – cutting, depression, severe anxiety, refusing to attend school. The first time I saw her I knew she was in need of counseling, preferably once per week. We made a referral for counseling, no appointments were available for over a month with anyone. This was not an option. After her second visit with me (one week later, she was not safe to have more time between visits) she decided that even if we could find a counselor for her, she did not want to go. She was not comfortable talking with anyone but me. Luckily, my practice was in a position at that time where I could see her weekly and provide talk therapy similar to what a counselor would have done. She is doing much better now and I see her beautiful smiling face monthly. We will be able to space that out even further very soon. The availability to spend 45 minutes to one hour weekly with a single child is not possible in a traditional pediatric practice. A pediatric mental health practice striving to deliver the best care must be able to provide counseling as needed, weekly or otherwise, for the health of our kids.

Chapter 4:

Cutting

The act of cutting is a symptom of an underlying problem. Kids do not pick up a sharp object such as a razor blade or hit a wall with such force to fracture a bone because they seek pain.

These types of behaviors are seen in all aspects of life. "Self-mutilation spares no social class. It spares no gender. It spares no ethnicity," says Dr. Armando Favazza (University of Missouri specializing in psychiatry and neurology with more than 50 years of experience in the field). The act of cutting has also been seen across time.

The first known documentation of self-cutting occurred in Ancient Greece and was recorded by Herodotus. The famous Greek historian wrote this about a Spartan leader who was imprisoned for his strange behavior. "And as he was lying there, fast bound, he noticed that all the guards had left him, except one, and he asked the man, who was his serf, to lend him his knife. As soon as the knife was in his hands, he began to mutilate himself, beginning on his shins." (1)

One big question – is self-harm innate or is it a learned behavior? Having historical references of self-injurious behavior from ancient Greece and then on through history makes one think this is possibly innate. It's something certain people just know how to do to relieve or distract from severe suffering. But, the significant increase in the behaviors over the past decade and the stories from children and adults who have tried self-harm shifts the thought to it possibly being a learned behavior as well. Regardless of origin, the physiologic response in the body to cutting is its own type of reward system.

The act of cutting causes a release of dopamine which is the feel-good neurotransmitter. It is self-reinforcing and can become extremely addictive. (2)

Children begin cutting for a number of reasons. Many times, they themselves do not understand why.

Depression

One of the symptoms commonly associated with depression is loss of emotion or dampening of feelings. Physical sensations can also be affected. Children often say they don't feel anything at all. Cutting makes them feel, physical pain is better than nothing.

Sometimes the inner pain and suffering can be so great that the cutting is a distraction. By inflicting physical pain, the attention and focus is pulled away from the emotional distress and onto something tangible, concrete. The cut is something they can see, feel, and process for what it is. Where feelings of internal pain which they do not typically understand and cannot process or improve is overwhelming. Often, they feel no ability to change or affect the internal turmoil.

Lack of Control

It can also be that the child feels no control in their environment. This could be home or school or friendships. Cutting is completely under their control. They have the ability to choose what item they use, where they cut, how deep to cut, how many cuts and how to hide them, and how to share the experience.

Abuse

With abuse there can be so much emotional and physical pain, children can learn to dissociate. This is described as coming out of your body. Some say it is as if they are floating above and see what is happening from a distance. That way the pain inflicted by another is not felt, only observed. This state can become the safe space and sometimes it can be hard to return back into the body, especially the older you get. Some use cutting to bring themselves back from this dissociative state.

To Belong

Another way children may discover self-harm or begin the cutting behavior is due to exposure through social media. Some kids start cutting to find a way to feel they belong. There is a significant presence online of pro self-harm websites, videos, and blogs. These sites educate on how to make cuts, what implements to use, how it can make you feel better and how to hide the wounds. It is so very important to know what your child is viewing and participating in online. Awareness of what is out there and then having open communication between child and parent is important in order to discuss the information seen online. The concepts and ideas portrayed online about self-harm can be overwhelming and hard to process for children. This may be just as true for the parent as well. Both parent and child need to recognize when using social media and the internet there is a good chance a child will be exposed to these ideals. Your child needs to feel comfortable coming to you to talk if they have questions or to simply talk about what has been seen.

Why Kids Don't Tell Their Parents

No matter how it begins, once the cutting starts, it tends to continue. This need to cut is often described as an urge. There is a lack of understanding about why it is happening for the children who participate. They know there is an emotional pain and that the cutting makes it better, then it becomes an urge which becomes something they cannot resist. This feels shameful in many ways.

Many kids who cut rarely share the occurrences with anyone, especially their parents. It is a very private thing and can become nearly ritualistic. For some, it is always the same sharp object such as a specific type of razor blade, done in the bathroom with the door locked, the cuts happening on the left wrist or ankles. They also may fear being judged by others. This is a process they cannot control which tends to escalate. The cuts can evolve becoming more frequent and deeper to get the sensation needed. This is a scary process which feels out of the child's control even if it started as a measure to gain some control of their environment.

Getting in Trouble

The fear of being in trouble is another reason many children will not tell anyone. If they do not understand why they do this, how could anyone else?

Not a Big Deal

Some children do not see cutting as a problem. It is seen on all forms of social media, in movies, and on TV. Friends have tried it. So, why does it matter?

Protecting the Parent

Then something I see often, is that the children try to protect their parents. Children know that when they are hurt, their parents get upset. A child believes if mom sees the marks on her arm, mom would cry or blame herself.

Children do not want a parent to blame themselves or be in pain because of something they did.

How to Talk to a Child Who Has Cut

For whatever reason, if a child chooses not to share their behavior with their parent, and then the parent finds out, all the parent wants to know is why. How did my child even know how to do this?

As the physician, I avoid asking why. Parents should avoid this question as well. "Why" puts children on the spot as if they should know and it makes it seem they are to blame, which is not true. In a straightforward, non-emotional manner, I ask if the child sitting with me has tried cutting. The first time I ask, they have a look of utter shock on their faces. Being upfront, open, and honest about a topic which is typically shunned is a surprise for them. I can see them process the question and then most of them will look me straight in the eye and say yes or no. For many, this is the first time they have admitted to cutting to anyone. They are able to answer because I ask the question just as all other questions are asked. Just as I ask about how are you sleeping? How has your appetite been? I ask all of my kids about it. Whether they are there for anxiety, depression, or any other concern. When they share, I have no reaction. There is no surprise, no worry or concern, no condemnation. It is, in fact, another piece of information we need to explore in the process of getting well.

Discovery Versus Disclosure

Typically, cutting behavior is discovered in a family rather than being disclosed spontaneously. It is rare for a child who has begun cutting to feel comfortable coming to a parent or family member and telling them outright.

One of my patients who I had been seeing for two weeks only, came in and sat down seeming happier than she had been during our two previous visits. She told me that she was working with her father on a project in the garage. Her sleeve shifted up on her arm and he saw her cuts. He exploded with anger. She then told him how she was feeling. She told him about the cutting, how long she had been doing it. She shared how deep her depression was and that she was having suicidal thoughts. She had never devised a specific plan on how she would take her life, but had suffered with that horrible, nagging feeling of not wanting to be present on the planet. Her father was able to calm himself and listen to her. He then made her go tell her mother. She went through the entire explanation once again. She was describing this to me and smiling. She was happy that they finally knew what she was going through and, as a result, she felt their relationship was better. She was then able to process her feelings from a place of stability which gave her perspective into the social dynamics of her family. These had been a significant contributor to her depressive state. Her depression is now under control and we are working on her anxiety. While she still sometimes feels the urge to cut, she now has tools in place to avoid the practice and has not cut in a significant amount of time.

There is no blame for cutting. It is an action which is initiated for as many reasons as there are individuals on this planet. It is scary for parents. It is not the parent's fault, or in any way, under their control. Every parent who discovers cuts on their child is shocked and cannot avoid the immediate thought of "what did I do wrong that my daughter would purposefully cut her skin?" As a parent, that thought cannot be avoided. It is innate. But, let me reassure you, you did not do this. Now all that matters is what you do going forward. What are the next steps you take? You will be told by every medical professional and counselor to make the home safe. Yes, this is important. But, know if your child has developed cutting behavior, no matter how many razors you hide, she will find an implement to cut when the urge hits. This is again not her fault and not yours. The underlying issue which has prompted her to cut must be ferreted out and treated. It is important to be open and honest. She must feel confident in her place in your heart to be able to come to you and say I am feeling the urge to cut and know you will not judge, or cry, or freak out. Patient support and appropriate individualized treatment will lay a new path over time for her to break the habit and stop cutting. This behavior is not your child's fault and is not the parents' fault. It is a symptom just like sadness and poor appetite. We treat the underlying cause, whatever it may be, and the symptom decreases and hopefully goes away completely.

Chapter 5:

A Child's Brain

When babies are born, they function on a system of need. There are no wants as we see them. They need food, comfort, and security. The newborn reflexes are to suck, grasp, and cry when feeling discomfort. They are hardwired once born to focus on a caregiver's face. This is how they first begin to learn about their world.

The concept of emotions as we understand them does not begin for children until later in life. The first year they respond to the emotions of others, begin to self soothe, and learn what behaviors elicit actions from the people around them. Games such as peek-a-boo, fake crying, and fake choking emerge during this time and train the adults very well.

Toddlers continue to evolve by learning through observing the emotions of their family and caregivers. They begin to become aware of their feelings and recognize that certain actions can cause emotional responses. It is a cause-and-effect system. A big spider jumping off the wall onto the floor near me scares me therefore I cry and run to mom who will protect me. This concept of perceived danger followed by rational fear of the danger and seeking comfort is how we as adults understand and interpret the scenario. For the child it is a physical response to the situation which they do not perceive as emotion or concept with a name. It is simple – heart rate jumps, blood pressure and breathing increase – seek comfort.

The child at preschool age begins to understand certain situations will elicit certain feelings - cause and effect. A hug from mom feels safe. A fall off the slide is scary. Rewards are given when I use good manners at the dinner table. Taking a cookie when told not to results in time-out. (3)

It is only in elementary school that kids begin to better label emotions and understand the concept that my feelings are not the same as yours. Even in this developmental stage it is very difficult for them to name the emotion. This becomes even more challenging when they feel the physiological response tied to emotion in a situation especially if it is powerful. We can recognize pride, shame, guilt, anger in their behaviors, but they cannot label their feelings as such. Children participate in interactions with others or their environment, have a physical response then act. So when you ask your competent, confident six-year-old why he smacked his two-year-old sister on the head while she was sleeping in her car seat. He will most likely respond "I don't know" and be 100% correct. He has absolutely no idea why. As adults we may see that he was bored and in need of attention or excitement, or she was sleeping on the toy he wanted, or she was blocking his view out of the window. For him it was an urge and he acted.

This concept applies to many behaviors and extends into middle school and then adolescence. In middle school, they develop the understanding that a person can have more than one feeling about another person. They begin to be capable of better identifying their own emotions. But still may not be able to put into words what emotions were felt, from where they came, and why those emotions caused an action or behavior. (4) An example would be a fifth-grade boy who sat in school all day on a day full of sunshine perfect to be outside playing, got a bad grade on a test, and the girl he likes took his milk at lunch. He goes to baseball practice and the coach is hard on the team and makes them run laps. Once he's back home, he sees that dinner is a new vegetarian pasta dish with tomatoes. He hates tomatoes. Before bed, dad comes in to put up his baseball glove and ball. He throws the baseball at the mirror and breaks it. Dad says, "Why did you throw the ball at the mirror?" His child says, "I don't know." He cannot process that he has had multiple frustrations during his day and that he has built up anger. All he knows is he feels horrible and lashes out.

This is a similar process with teenagers who feel strong emotions. A bad day at school with poor friend interactions brings emotional pain which then causes them to react by skipping basketball practice after school. They have a hard time labeling the emotions as sadness, frustration, betrayal, anger. In order to process emotions, they need to first be identified. Once identified and named, they become tangible and therefore can be responded to with conscious actions/behaviors.

This evolution in emotional processing is seen in the brain's physical growth and development along with the emergence of executive function. Per Russell Barkley, PhD, "executive function is defined as self-regulation across time for the attainment of one's goals (long-term self-interests) typically in the context of others and often using social and cultural means." (5) Executive function is attained with the development/maturation of the right pre- frontal cortex. This area of the brain becomes mature sometime in the twenties depending on genetics and upbringing. This is important because a significant piece of executive function is self- regulation of emotion. If this does not develop until at least twenty years of age, how do we expect our children to name, process, and respond to a highly charged often unreliable environment. This is beautifully stated by Dr. Barkley in his CME course titled: "Executive Functioning: Nature, Assessment, and Management" last revised 11-14-18.

Self-Regulation of Emotion

"Often overlooked in cold cognitive accounts of executive function (EF), yet prolific in the description of various disorders of the pre-frontal cortex (PFC), is the inability to self-regulate strong emotions that may be elicited by environmental events yet which are not in the longer-term best self-interests of the individual to display. Raw emotional displays, unmodified as to their appropriateness to a given social context, and poorly moderated as to the longer-term adverse social impact they are likely to have is a recipe for impaired social relationships if not outright rejection by others. Humans possess a means by which they can inhibit the initial displays of strong emotions and subsequently engage in a series of actions that suppress, modify, and otherwise moderate the eventual expression of the emotion so that it is more socially acceptable and consistent with the individual's longer-term goals and welfare. This is believed to be achieved by the bi-directional network of connections among the dorsolateral frontal cortex, orbital-frontal cortex, anterior cingulated cortex, and amygdala (and hence limbic system). Such a system permits not merely the self-regulation of elicited emotion but the conscious and volitional *utilization* of emotional states in the service of a person's goals and longer-term welfare. Emotions become experiences that are not merely provoked and therefore must be subsequently dealt with appropriately but are also states that can be created *de novo* as needed in the service of one's goals."

So what does this mean? How do I talk to my child about her emotions? Regardless of age, the key is to not ask why. They may not know. They may have some understanding but do not have the words or they may not want to say. Asking concrete questions about a specific behavior can help a child begin to name what they were feeling in the moment then start understanding emotion.

For example our little boy from above who had a bad day and threw his baseball breaking the mirror in his room.

One version of the conversation could be:

Dad: Why did you do that?

Boy: I don't know

Dad: What do you mean you don't know? You broke your mirror.

Boy (Now crying): I don't know.

Dad (Now yelling): How could you do this?

Boy (No longer answering): ...

Version two:

Dad: What happened?

Boy: I threw the ball.

Dad: What were you thinking about right before you threw the ball?

Boy: I don't know

Dad: OK, then what was your body feeling?

Boy: My head was hurting, my eyes were stingy, and my chest felt hot.

Dad: What were you thinking about before you came in your room and felt your head hurting and your chest hot? My body can feel that way when I am mad.

Boy: Coach is mean.

Dad: What happened during baseball practice?

Boy: We had to run laps, but I didn't do anything wrong. I hate math....

Dad: What happened in school today?

Boy: I got a bad grade and Ashley stole my milk at lunch.

Dad: What did your body feel like when those things happened?

Etc....

This process opens a dialogue in which the boy can link the situations in his day to how he was feeling and then possibly to his actions in the moment of anger. Where the first example will just cause frustration and hurt for both dad and his son.

Each step in the conversation is to be small, manageable, and without blame. Asking about actions and physical sensations which are concrete therefore easy to express in words.

Always work back in time. If he is unable to say what he was thinking or feeling before an incident, you can then try specific physical sensations. Such as "what was your head feeling?"

If he is not able to identify his thoughts for the moment in question, go back farther in time more with "What were you thinking before we came into your room?" This process allows him to follow his thoughts through time and then link them to physical sensations which can then link to emotions.

You may have to help name the emotion by restating whatever he says. Such as: "You said you were thinking about all the bad things in your day, your head felt full, your stomach hurt, and your heart was beating fast then you threw the ball. That sounds like anger to me."

You can also use colors for reference. Feelings of anger are sometimes associated with the color red. Happiness can be yellow, pink, or associated with the sensation of being warm. Sadness can be blue. If words are hard, use a white board or paper with crayons to express thoughts and feelings. There are no limits to how you approach this. Use your own creativity and what you know about how your child likes to engage.

The conversation should be age appropriate including length. A six-year-old can work through this process for 5-10 minutes maximum, where a teenager could participate for 20-30 minutes (depending on their emotional state and interest). This process does not work when in the height of emotion. Think of a time when you with your fully developed frontal cortex had an emotional explosion. Could you think logically in any way? Neither can our kids.

A perfect example of this process is a fifteen-year-old female patient of mine. She was struggling with why she had an explosive, emotional fight with her grandmother which resulted in her depression relapsing and cutting. We sat and talked through the events leading up to her relapse. She could not remember what her grandmother said which made her so angry. So, we went a step back. She had just come home from track. She is a sprinter and was working on her splits for the 440-yard dash. She missed her goal time on each of four tries. She stated that made her really angry; she felt as if she failed herself. After further conversation about the goals she set for her splits, those times were the goals set for her reach by the end of the season. They had just started practicing, it was the very beginning of track season. She realized her anger at herself was probably more than it should have been and not how she would normally have responded in that situation. So, we went back farther in her day. Just prior to track practice, she and her boyfriend had a really big fight. When asked, she admitted that the fight started over him wanting to give her a ride home after track so she did not have to walk. She was so frustrated she had considered breaking up with him. After talking about the event with me when not in the throes of the emotions which were happening at that time, she again was able to see that her level of anger with him was not how she would have normally reacted in that situation. So we walked further back in time to the previous day. That day had been hard, she was tired, and had done poorly on a test. Then she remembered running into her father who she rarely sees at a coffee shop. He saw her but turned his back and walked out with his new family. He did not acknowledge or speak to her. Her eyes became wide and she saw clearly the series of events for what they were. She then could process how each emotion was a reaction to a specific event and then transmuted causing her to react in a way she would not typically do and then to act out in ways that were not normal behaviors for her. In the height of the moment she could not name her feelings much less process them in order to manage them to change the outcome which was her cutting relapse. The exercise of talking through the events going back in time gave her clarity in hindsight. So the next time a scenario begins to unfold she can identify each step for what it is and address the negative response or emotion in the beginning to avoid the end consequence or behavior.

Emotional dysregulation can be an early sign of both depression and anxiety. Depression is rooted in sadness where anxiety is rooted in fear. Both are mediated and affected by the chemical neurotransmitters in the brain.

Chapter 6:

Pathophysiology

Cutting is a symptom not a diagnosis. It does not stand on its own. It is a behavior caused by or born out of an underlying condition. It is not caused by parenting or a choice children make. It is not a behavior a parent can say, "Stop or I will punish you by taking your phone." It is not that simple. It is not within the behaviors parents have the power to stop through discipline. It is an action based upon a neurochemical imbalance in the brain which can be secondary to a variety of mental health conditions. In other words, the brain chemistry has been changed in some way so it is not working well. This is the most common cause of mental illnesses. These conditions can be depression, anxiety, history of trauma, ADHD, etc. It is also commonly a combination of these. To treat and heal, the correct cause needs to be determined. If a child is cutting due to depression and the focus of treatment is on trauma which she does not consider a part of her concerns, she will not improve. Accurate diagnosis is imperative to treatment and therefore healing.

In addition to a correct diagnosis, the treatment must also be chosen with the understanding and knowledge that each child is different. They are biochemically and developmentally unique. In addition, while being treated over time their individual needs can evolve. The treatment may start focused on ADHD then change over to or include treatment for anxiety. A concern with diagnosis is that the symptoms which are present in children can be similar between the various causes. A child with ADHD may be exhibiting behavior which has the parent convinced they are suffering from profound anxiety. This is a pattern I see often. I will have a consult for a six-year-old girl for anxiety referred to me by their primary care provider. After taking the time to complete a full evaluation the child is diagnosed with ADHD and treatment started. The symptoms mimic one another. The symptoms which manifest are the result of the neurotransmitters in the brain.

In theory, each diagnosis has a specific neurotransmitter or neurotransmitter imbalance associated with it. Depression is traditionally associated with serotonin. Anxiety is associated with norepinephrine. Schizophrenia is associated with dopamine. Mood disorders can involve all three. This is an extremely simplistic picture to make it understandable to us all. There are currently greater than 100 identified neurotransmitters. More are being discovered all the time. You will find references which state greater than 200 have been identified. I like to describe the neurotransmitter pool as a bowl of vegetable soup. There are many ingredients, each has a place and function. But we aren't completely sure how each spice or vegetable contributes to the overall end-result. We do know what role the carrots, onions, and potatoes play. According to Dr. Stephen Stahl, there are six key neurotransmitter systems which should be focused on in diagnosis and treatment, primarily because they have been well-researched and are affected by the current medications used. These are serotonin, norepinephrine, dopamine, acetylcholine, glutamate, and GABA – our carrots, potatoes, and onions. (6)

Our focus is on cutting and its cause and how to treat it. Understanding depression, one of the most common underlying processes associated with cutting, is a must. The nervous system is made up of cells called neurons. They do not touch one another but must communicate to function. They use chemistry and electricity to achieve this. A signal is passed from one end of an individual neuron to the other by an electrical impulse. Once it hits the end of that particular cell, the signal must be passed onto the next one by other means. This is done by the neurotransmitters. The small gap between each neuron is called a synapse. The electrical impulse comes to the end of the neuron and depending on what the intended signal is a neurotransmitter is released into the synapse to carry that message onto the next cell. So now the signal can move on and carry its message onto the next cell or other intended target.

The neurotransmitters are held in little bubbles called vesicles until they are needed to be released. When released, they cross the gap and either stimulate the next cell's electrical impulse, stop an action of the next cell, slow down or speed up a process or affect organs to respond in certain ways. Once the neurotransmitter has done its job by causing something to occur in the next cell, the cell sucks it back into its vesicles through reuptake channels which are regulated by transporters, enzymes, and receptors. Some neurotransmitters stay in the synapse rather than being held in vesicles. The overriding theory with depression is that the levels of serotonin that are supposed to stay in the synapse have become low. This can be caused by stress, genetic predisposition, lack of sleep, trauma. The unfortunate process with this is that the symptoms of depression such as lack of sleep create a vicious cycle. The symptom itself causes the serotonin levels to become more diminished which, in turn, increases the symptoms making the depression worse. A child who has experienced a trauma, such as a best friend who is diagnosed with cancer, gets really worried about his friend. That worry eats up a bit of serotonin in his synapses. So now he has a harder time falling asleep and he's getting less sleep each night. The lack of sleep now eats more of the available serotonin which should be hanging out in the synapse. Now the serotonin levels are even lower causing even worse sleep patterns which then lead to more symptoms of low serotonin.

The synaptic concentration of neurotransmitters can be described as bumper cars. If there are many in a group when one comes forward and hits the first one in the group, that physical bump or energy is felt all the way to the other end by the first hitting the second the second then hitting the third, and so on. This is what happens with neurotransmitters. If there are not enough present in the synapse when the signal is released the signal just stops. There are not enough cars to get the signal across the synapse to its destination and produce the intended effect. This equates to feelings of sadness, lack of motivation, poor appetite, lack of feeing, lack of focus. When in this state, a child is more likely to have associated feelings of fear which can lead to anxiety symptoms as well. Stressors affect our brain's neurochemistry.

The bathtub model is a good, real world example of how our bodies process and can cope with stress. We look at our body as a bathtub which holds all our emotions and thoughts. There is the big white tub, the faucet, and the drain. Stress comes in from the faucet and goes out through the drain. If the drain is plugged and the faucet continues to run the tub will fill. If that continues, the tub will fill and then overflow. This is the state where an outburst, cutting or other harmful behaviors occur. At all times, our aim should be to prevent an overflow, to maintain our tub in a state where it cannot overflow. What is under an individual's control is what comes in and what goes out. We have the ability to turn off the faucet or open the drain and release some of the water. To control what comes in and what is let out is something which has must be learned. It is not natural. For children, they do not understand their bathtub. They do not understand what emotion is, much less how to attend to certain ones and disregard others (turning off the faucet.) They do not have the capacity to look at an emotion such as getting in trouble at school for something they did not do, see it as not their fault, accept that the teacher made a mistake, and then choose an appropriate response to the situation. For the child, the choices could be (1) talk to the teacher and explain the situation so she understands it was not his doing or (2) accept that the teacher was in error but she is working very hard in a classroom of 30 children and it was not a slight specifically against him. Either scenario would allow him to release the emotion from his bathtub by resolving the situation in his own mind through perspective. But children feel the physical symptoms of anger and frustration, cannot necessarily name them, do not have executive function to assess the situation to gain perspective and then resolve the conflict for themselves. Therefore, they cannot unplug and release anything. So the small tub gets full and the only release is action in some form, typically an acting out behavior.

This jump to action can also be consistent with anxiety. The feeling of anxiety is best understood by looking at the fight or flight reflex. Our hind brain (caveman or reptilian brain), the oldest part of our brain, is run strictly on survival. When something happens this part of the brain assesses the situation and decides if it is a threat. Once threat status is established, it launches fight or flight where your nervous system is primed for one action or the other. Either way – heart rate goes up, respiratory rate goes up, blood is diverted from organs to the muscles. This can be accompanied with headaches, nausea, abdominal pain, and dizziness. Or as we call it today, panic. It is complete, full on activation of the sympathetic nervous system. The problem is that in our modern world we are not having to run from cave lions in order to survive or fight the caveman next-door for the safety of our family. Our brains can perceive or interpret common life events as threats. A teacher getting mad for something I did not do. My boyfriend talking with his ex. My parents arguing, again. Once activated, this mechanism can stay primed, therefore more likely to activate again with less of a trigger. We see this with kids who have been exposed to domestic violence or have been abused. This activation affects neurotransmitters and can lead to imbalances. These imbalances can then be reflected in the behaviors and symptoms we see.

As fight or flight is one specific pathway in the brain which launches due to an event creating a response, there are millions of other pathways also present. I like to describe this best as a roadmap. Anyone who has been to Portland, Oregon can relate well. On a map, there are roads going in all different directions. Some are straight, many are small and curved. There are different paths to get to the same place. The brain is the same. When we are born the brain consists of billions of interconnections, different pathways to arrive at the same conclusion. As we age and gain experiences and learn, some pathways are selected as preferred. As these pathways are used more and more, they develop from windy dirt roads to two-lane paved streets and, over time, to huge eight-lane superhighways. This works the same for thoughts, emotions, and actions.

When the superhighway is built these pathways are now akin to habits. You have a starting point, an emotion, event, even scent, and all of a sudden you end up at the action without experiencing the path. For example, you smell the chocolate chip cookies your next-door neighbor is cooking and find yourself on grandmother's porch. Grandma baked the best cookies, and this is a strong memory. But you did not notice gathering your belongings, getting in the car, driving to the highway, setting the car on cruise for 20 miles, driving into her town, parking in her drive, getting out of the car, and walking up the steps. This is the same process which can happen in a child's brain. They are told "no" about playing video games and end up in a tantrum kicking the walls. Or, a teenager gets looked at with perceived judgment, across a classroom by a person who was her friend and she goes into the bathroom and cuts her arm with the razor blade she keeps with her. All they recognize is a physical sensation and an action is taken, not the many steps between. It has become automatic.

Another aspect is impulsivity. Children have not developed those executive function skills of assessing a situation and then making a choice between available actions. This is a slightly different way to get from an external influence to action compared to the highway or pathway analogy. Children are naturally impulsive. But this is also compounded by ADHD. ADHD, like other mental health diagnosis, is modulated by neurotransmitters, mainly dopamine and norepinephrine. ADHD is typically characterized by inability to focus, impulsivity, overactivity, and unpredictability. Children with ADHD tend to have problems with motivation, staying on task, short-term memory, and control of their emotions. It can be difficult for them to participate in games and sports. When distractible a child tends to miss part of the instructions but even if you got the rules you might miss a step in the actual play. It also leads to difficulty functioning within a classroom. If you do not hear all the rules, how do you participate as expected?

This missing out on information is not the child's fault. The ADHD brain functions differently than those without ADHD. The inability to participate as expected in social settings can lead to sadness, rejection, anger, and frustration which, of course, they perceive at their level of development as physical sensations they often cannot name or process. The inability to understand the rules of social engagement can also lead to fear of situations. If you don't know how to behave and keep getting in trouble for something you do not understand, you develop fear which can lead to or look like anxiety.

The aspect of impulse control is especially important to understand in our children. A thought enters their heads and unfiltered it comes out their mouths or an action is taken. A patient of mine is the perfect example. This darling seven-year-old girl who was beloved by her classmates and teachers kept getting into trouble at school. She picked up the nearest phone and called 911 when her best friend asked her what would happen if they called that number. She released the class pet hamster into the school hallway so it could be free. She pulled the fire alarm to see how loud it really was - all behaviors mediated by lack of impulse control. The thought entered her mind and she took immediate action without the ability to consider there might be consequences for her, her friends, or the hamster. If she had the ability to assess what might happen due to those impulses, she probably would not have gone through with any of them. This impulsivity also affects the actions of self-harm. A child with ADHD, when down would be more likely to try cutting for the first time because they saw how it made someone feel better on a video or read about it online. They do not stop to consider what they are doing or what could happen next.

Cutting is a symptom and can be caused or influenced by so many aspects of a child's life. The physiology of a child's brain makes them even more vulnerable to this behavior. Depression, anxiety, ADHD are all conditions caused by an imbalance in neurotransmitters in the brain and can lead to self-harm. Each of these diagnoses can begin with a genetic predisposition. All tend to run in families, but that does not mean a child cannot develop one of these conditions if there is no family history present. More often than not, we cannot pinpoint a single cause of a child's depression or anxiety. And we cannot predict which child with one of these conditions will cut. What matters is that it is a chemical function, not a temperament, or choice, or just a bad kid. Understanding how the brain works and that it is not the child's or parent's fault is the best place to begin to move forward and work on recovery.

Chapter 7:

Treatment

Through history treatment of mental health problems has been structured around the goal of a partial reduction in symptoms. With depression, it was considered a treatment success if symptoms were reduced by 50 percent. This paradigm, thank goodness, has shifted with now a goal of complete remission. This, I believe, is even more important with children. Their brains are continuing to develop. They require input and experience to begin to understand their emotions then to regulate them. They must have the ability to pay attention in class to learn not only schoolwork but the rules of social interaction. They need structure and reinforcement in appropriate behaviors. They need the education and exposure to techniques which can help them learn to first understand what they are feeling, process that feeling, and then choose how they wish to respond to that feeling. To be able to learn the multitude of techniques available and to find what works for you requires that your brain has the capability to hear, take in, then understand the lesson. This requires that the lesson be presented in a developmentally appropriate manner and that the brain has the neurotransmitter balance to be present.

A severely depressed child who has not been sleeping well or eating properly for months and who has started cutting will not be able to process a counseling session about letting go of negative emotions. It would be similar to being taught how to prepare the perfect beef stroganoff over the phone by someone who only speaks an unknown foreign language and then being held responsible by your family for the dish not turning out right.

Medication

The medications we have today are a useful tool to help balance neurotransmitters and provide a platform for other therapies to be effective. I do not believe all children need medications to heal, but if needed they can be safe and effective when used properly. In many children, we use the Specific Serotonin Reuptake Inhibiter (SSRI) class of medications for depression and anxiety which have been on the market for more than 25 years. Also used are medications which will have some effect on norepinephrine and serotonin in the synapse. There are specific norepinephrine reuptake inhibitors (SNRIs) available as well which can be helpful in anxiety and work for some with ADHD. Stimulants are used for ADHD and have been around for seventy years.

The SSRIs work on the neurotransmitter at the synapse. [NSRI, norepinephrine and serotonin reuptake inhibitors and SNRI, specific norepinephrine reuptake inhibitor, medications work along the same principle. When the signal comes down the nerve causing the serotonin to be released from the vesicle into the synapse, the serotonin crosses the synapse to pass on its message to the next neuron. The goal of these medications is to increase the amount of neurotransmitter in the synapse. The lack of available serotonin is what causes the symptoms we associate with depression – sadness, lack of motivation, agitation, guilt, sleep, and appetite disturbances. The increase in neurotransmitter volume occurs by the medication blocking the cells' normal pattern of pulling the serotonin out of the synapse after it has completed passing on the intended signal. This allows the serotonin to build back up to normal levels in the synapse.

The SSRIs are a large class of medications. They primarily affect serotonin but have subtle differences from one another. Each medicine affects a specific receptor which moves the serotonin from the synapse into a vesicle, but then they have additional receptors which can have an effect on the uptake of other neurotransmitters as well. Sertraline, for instance, has some mild effect on dopamine as well as serotonin. Different medications will affect norepinephrine in addition to serotonin or perhaps another of the neurotransmitters.

The complexity of the medications used to treat depression or anxiety is one of the reasons why it is important to know the education and experience of the person who is treating your child. Many feel comfortable using only one specific medication at low doses. This does not translate to healing. Each child is an individual with a unique brain which has been affected by their experience, genetics, and circumstance. One medication is not going to help all children. As stated before, the correct diagnosis is required first then an appropriate medication is chosen then tailored to the child. The doses are adjusted or the medication changed based upon how symptoms are responding to the treatment. Due to the way the medications rebuild the serotonin supply in the synapse, they often take time to work. First, it will typically be the close family who sees an improvement in mood or level of interaction. This can occur two to three weeks after starting one of the SSRIs. The child will begin to feel a bit more energetic, then mood improves at three to four weeks. The full effect of the medicine is not known until they have been taking it for approximately six weeks. Monitoring and supporting through this time are very important and should be taken very seriously by your prescriber.

Using medications in the treatment of depression, anxiety, or any other cause for cutting is not mandated or always necessary. The choice to use medications should follow a thoughtful discussion which occurs between parent, child, and doctor. Choosing to start medications does not mean a failure on any person's part or that you are taking the easy way out. Medications are a tool specifically used to balance the brain's chemistry in order for the other modalities of treatment to be effective. A trial of an antidepressant be it for depression or anxiety is exactly that, a trial.

Medications are metabolized differently in children versus adults. The doses may be different and will need adjustment. Once medications are started there is an ongoing dialogue about how the child is responding. Changes are made to ensure the optimal outcome. The dose may need changed. The medication may need to be a different one in the same class or a medication in a different class may be a better fit. When treating depression, once the medication which matches the needs for the specific brain chemistry of your child is found (it works for them), the medication should be continued for approximately six months. The reasoning is that it takes time for the brain to adjust and balance. If symptoms have resolved and the appropriate time has passed, we then wean the medication off slowly. This is done to allow the body to take over the action which was being provided by the medication. If done properly, the brain has adjusted and now can maintain the appropriate balance of neurotransmitters in the synapse without medication support. This also decreases significantly the chance of a relapse. If the medication is stopped without a wean, there can be side effects. These do not damage the brain, but it may make the child feel bad. They can have headaches, body aches, and feel over or under stimulated. Stopping the medicine suddenly also increases the likelihood the depression and associated symptoms will come right back. Stopping medication against medical advice is something encountered often during treatment for a variety of reasons.

Family and cultural background play a big part in treatment or non-treatment of any mental illness. I have a 15-year-old boy as a patient who suffers with depression and anxiety. He is of Latino descent. There is an element of Latino culture that suggests it is a weakness for men to have mental health concerns. Medications are frowned upon and counseling is not an option. We have been working together for six months and this young man always came in alone. His family was not participating in his care or treatment plan. We met three times before he was able to share his whole story which included some significant trauma. He agreed to medication and took it as prescribed for one month. He felt a bit better and stopped. I saw him again. He shared he had stopped his medication. We went through how and why the medicine works again. He decided not to restart even though he was still having significant depressive symptoms. It was his decision, I cannot make him take medications, just share my recommendations based upon his history and current condition. A month later, he returned and started meds again because his symptoms had worsened. He stopped them on his own once again after about a month because he was feeling better and his family was against him taking anything. They felt he should be able to tough it out. We discussed that he was not helping his brain recover and I did not prescribe more of the SSRI. If it is not being used as it should be, it is no longer a useful tool which can add to his recovery. My belief that his brain would benefit greatly from the medication became irrelevant due to the situation. He had already had some success but could not follow the plan to take his medications as prescribed. He will begin counseling soon even against the cultural bias. I have to wonder where he could be today if he had family support.

Medications are a tool to support brain function so that the harder work of education and counseling can begin. One goal of treatment is to teach a child to get off their highway - that immediate response to a stimulus which has been trained into their brain. Medications can slow down anxiety and the jump to fight or flight. They can help in stabilizing appetite and sleep or increase motivation. But the ability to understand and name emotions, then react to the same stimulus in a different way, takes work. I teach my kids this analogy. They understand that the highway is present and for their behavior to change they must find ways to kick themselves off. We sometimes say, "take the closest exit." In order to do this the first thing is to work through what their trigger is. It could be anything in their environment, a situation, a specific feeling, a person, a place, or date. Once it or they have been identified, recognizing when you encounter your trigger is imperative. The next step is seeing the highway and where it leads. It could lead to cutting, to crying, to withdrawing, to punching a wall, or other people. That knowledge in and of itself is powerful. But the task is to get off the highway between the stimulus and the action occurs best initially through distraction. The best distraction includes engagement of the mind, body, and emotions. Each child has to figure out their own distraction. What works for one individual will not work for another. Some will choose more than one. One to do in public and one in private. It does not matter what it is, only that it works for them.

Experimenting with different distraction activities can be entertaining and something you can do with your child. It can be as simple as having a worry stone or other object in their pocket. When triggered they rub the stone and count backward from ten in a foreign language. Another option is to do five jumping jacks while singing your favorite song. It does not need to last but a few seconds. The idea is to break the pattern. The first time is hardest. It gets easier and easier as the worn path is averted. There are also specific tools to respond to the urge to cut such as snapping a band on the wrist or using ice in the place of a sharp object to mimic pain with another sensation.

Breathing

A good tool is 1:2 breathing. It is very calming for the nervous system and can be a distractor as well. For this, you breathe in a set number of your choice, say two, three, or four. Then breathe out double that number. So, if you breathe in for three, the exhale would be six. Another technique is box breathing. This literally creates a square. Set a number and breathe for that count. Say you choose four. Breathe in for the count of four, then hold that breath for the count of four, breathe out for four then hold your breath for another count of four. I think this works best for teenagers and for physical pain. There is an array of breathing techniques out there. It could be a fun game to research the options with your child and then test them out together.

There will be one or two that resonate with your child. Once that something has been selected, practice when not in crisis. You have to develop the feel of it and be able to perform the technique when calm before it can be used when needed. A good practice is to do it before bed. It can be added into a bedtime routine and done together or even as a group. The more they get used to the calming effect, the better it can help when the time comes.

Peripheral Focusing

The act of focusing on peripheral vision when added to a calming breathing technique is extremely effective. This can be used in school age and up. You sit calmly and begin your choice of breathing. Then pick a place to focus on in the distance straight in front of you. For younger kids help them choose a specific item on which to focus. When learning this relaxation tool, do it with your child. Together you can make it a game. Fix your vision on a chosen object in front of you then relax your eyes a bit to take notice of the items present in your peripheral vision. You can then play I-spy with the objects in peripheral vision while keeping your eyes straight ahead toward the original object. As this is practiced, it becomes easier. It can be done without others being aware and is extremely de-excitatory for the nervous system.

Externalizing Focus

Another great distraction technique is to bring the focus from within to the external environment. A specific way to do this is to follow five, four, three, two, one. First look about and name five things you see. Next look around and name four things you could touch, then name three things you could hear, next name two things you could smell then one thing you could taste. This forces the brain to concentrate on or notice what is surrounding you in your environment. It is dealing with the five senses which are grounding and concrete so you can deescalate a high emotional state. This is also a practice which should be played with and practiced when not in crisis. It is much easier to learn a new tool when calm. It can be introduced just as another new type of I-Spy that you as a parent want to try. Sometimes saying you are going to learn a new calming technique will close a young mind to all ideas. Every new concept or trial of a technique should be light and fun. Your child will respond to some and not others. It is a process of trying on as many as needed until you find a comfortable fit. Hopefully there will be a few. The more tools in your tool bag the better.

Tapping

A favorite technique for many people is tapping. It's used in mainstream medicine and energy work. There are many variations, approaches, and uses. I teach the simplest version because it makes sense to the kids, is easy to use, and is effective. This is another to practice before the impulse or emotional crisis begins. One version is to lightly stamp your feet alternating. Tap right foot on the ground, left foot on the ground. Then keep repeating. It does not matter which side you start with. It is best done sitting. The gentle rhythmic impact can reset the nervous system just enough to get that split second to process information – to breathe – get off the highway. Another tapping exercise is to tap with your fingers on the outside of the thighs just above the knees. Again right, left, right, left. It works the same way and can be very relaxing. In an emotionally overwhelmed state, tapping with the three middle fingers repeatedly on the upper sternum (breastbone) can be relaxing and release some of that build-up of feelings.

Counseling

Counseling goes hand in hand with any mental health treatment in the pediatric population. The counselors work to teach kids techniques to get them through events such as breathing, alternative focus, and tapping described above. There is a multitude of techniques. Counselors are adept at finding ones that will fit with your child and work with their specific needs. But they also work much deeper and teach through varied therapies. They can work through the identification of emotions, the ability to choose how to respond, and what actions will be taken based upon emotion or stimulus. Common therapies include CBT (cognitive behavioral therapy), EMDR (Eye Movement and Desensitization and Reprocessing), DBT (Dialectical Behavioral Therapy), and many others. Each can be used for differing conditions or needs or ages. Most counselors will be trained in one or more techniques. Choose your counselor with care and research. There are many types with differing backgrounds, focus, and approaches.

Meditation

Meditation is an amazing tool which can be taught at a young age. There are books and some teachers who can assist in this. Coleman, an elementary school in

Baltimore, uses meditation and yoga in place of certain punishments. When children act out or need calming, they go to a mindfulness room where staff is available. They also go through breathing techniques and movement in the mornings as a school and prior to leaving. They are finding great improvements in behaviors and academics due to this practice. Other schools across the US are implementing mindfulness as a resource. (7)

Journaling

Journaling is one of my favorite techniques, and one my teenagers always roll their eyes at when I introduce it. My idea of journaling is not a diary where you write down every part of your day in detail. It's writing down anything that feels right at that moment. The act of putting pen to paper has a unique effect on the brain. The brain is composed of two hemispheres. One is in charge of primarily emotions and one is the analytical or thinking side. The sides connect across a thin band of tissue called the corpus collosum. When one side of the brain is overly active or activated, the interaction of the two sides across the corpus collosum is diminished, sometimes impossible. So when the emotional side is having crises with depression or anxiety the thinking side is not able to engage and provide perspective.

When you write, pen to paper, it improves communication between the hemispheres which helps you better understand. One of my young adult patients was in complete emotional crisis over a breakup with her long-term boyfriend. She was crying all the time, would not go to work or school, would not eat and was not sleeping. She tried journaling and discovered her sadness and grief was not over the guy specifically, which is what she was focused on, but rather it was the fear of the loss of companionship. She was afraid of being alone with high school graduation happening in a few weeks. This came out fairly quickly with the journaling and then we were able to address the fears. She then recovered without need for further interventions.

If angry, a child can color the entire page black with a pen. If happy, they can draw a smiley face and be done. If it feels right for them to write about their day and emotions, great, go for it. If they feel like writing poetry, a story, or a song, that is fabulous. They can draw a picture as simple or as detailed as they like. It does not matter. These pages are to be kept by the child, not by their parents, friends, counselor or doctor. It is private and for them personally, not other people. If they write about something they needed to get rid of, they can just tear out that page and shred it. With adult supervision, it can also be burned safely. They are only limited by their imagination. I recommend they do this every night before bed. We as humans use in the conscious state somewhere between 3 and 10 percent of our brains. The other 90+ percent is the subconscious. I believe that journaling prior to sleep can engage the subconscious, perhaps bringing even more clarity and perspective to the process.

Chapter 8:

Obstacles

This path to get help for your child is not an easy one. Unfortunately, there are many challenges to be faced. Once the discovery is made that your child has cut themselves, the flood gate is open. As a parent, you must choose to move beyond your own biases and expectations. How can my child have cut? This is something that happens to other families, not mine. Depression does not happen in children, what do they have to worry about? Uncle Frank committed suicide at age 20, is that what is going to happen? These are just few of the thoughts that can come up. The journey to health, happiness, and success for your child is colored by the belief systems within your culture, society, or family. The concerns do not just arise from the pre-conceived notions of the parents or extended family, but the children themselves will have just as many, if not more, reasons to resist treatment.

Once cutting has started there is a mark, a symptom that is tangible. It is out and all can see. But only if caught. I can hide what I am doing under my sleeves or pants. No one has to know. No one can know. What will they think of me? I can't tell them what I am doing. I can't explain to them why I do this. All I know is that I feel better afterward. Sometimes I can't remember a time without cutting. Sometimes I cannot remember a time I was happy. My friend who knows now what I have done, won't talk to me. Will my parents feel the same way? Will they be angry? Will they be sad and cry? I don't want my mom to cry. Will she blame herself? It was nothing she did or didn't do. It just is. Why do I hurt so much? Why can I not stop? No one could possibly understand. How could they understand? I don't understand. I don't feel anything. I am never hungry then I am starving. How can I be gaining weight? I am ugly now. How can anyone love me?

As a parent, you want to help your child but your words fall onto ears which cannot hear. Their minds are full of self-loathing, sadness, fear and guilt. How do you break through that dialogue to convince your child to get help? This is one of the hardest steps. It takes patience and perseverance. But it can be done.

Once you have broken through the hard shell your child erected and she has heard. Your concerns and hope for getting help have been acknowledged and finally your child says "okay, I will see someone." What is next? She refuses to go to a counselor. She will see the PA she sees for ear infections, but you know they are not qualified for this. What do you do? If she is willing to see a counselor because you have pressed the issue, how can you be sure she will talk? You can't. You can just get her there, be supportive, and hope it is a good fit. If the counselor does not connect with your child, what next? Move on. Find another. The most important piece is connection. Your child must feel comfortable and trust the person they are talking to about such personal moments. Moments they do not understand and are afraid to even see. Counseling is to look, understand, and accept so life can go on and flourish.

The next challenge is insurance. What do they pay for and why? Once you find a personality match for your child, what happens if they do not take your insurance. Or even, will insurance cover counseling at all? If not, how do I pay? How do I choose? There is no perfect answer to this. You may need to take some time to research and seek out other options, but it is important that you navigate the process.

The system itself, regulated by insurance companies and large corporations, is lacking in resources. There are too few doctors who have the needed knowledge. The doctors who want to help may not have enough time in their daily schedule. There are simply not enough pediatric psychiatrists available to consult or evaluate kids with severe crisis or more complex mental illnesses. There are not enough counselors trained to work with children. The institutions where children could get inpatient mental healthcare are full, or do not have enough staff or resources to care for those who are in need. Or, they cannot handle higher acuity. They have their limits and, if not available, it is just too bad. Families are left out on their own. The gaps between minor needs and crisis which leaves families alone and struggling are real.

There is also the gap in the medical profession due to provider discrimination. The doctors you see may not know anything about mental health. They may not like mental health as a profession. They may see children with mental health illness as faking or exaggerating. This is sad and unfortunate, but present in our system. If you encounter one of these, what do you do? How do you get past a gatekeeper to a person equipped and willing to help?

Navigating the system is hard enough, but what this does to the family unit is a piece rarely considered until you are living it. As a loving parent, there is no way to escape some sort of self-blame. I should have known something was wrong. It was something I did or did not do that brought us here to this point. This is a normal process, but there was no way for you to predict. Your child did not become anxious or depressed and begin cutting because you missed the last performance of a play or did not attend a soccer game or buy her the phone she wanted. Then once the flood gates are open, communication suffers. A child is still struggling to understand for themselves and cannot share what is happening inside out of fear from judgement, causing further pain. As the parent you become overly sensitive to her moods. You stop disciplining out of fear of causing further cutting or worsening depression. You feel as if you are walking on eggshells all the time and no longer know how to function in your own home. Every waking minute is to be on high alert, watching for signs of worsening condition, mood, or injury. This takes a toll on everyone. It uses up the parents' energy. There is nothing left to give to dad, the siblings, even the dog. This can create discord. Parents begin to struggle in their relationship. There are disagreements about treatment options, money, how to discipline, how to manage time between home, school, work, doctors' appointments, extracurricular activities for your other kids. Life changes from proactive participation to defensive survival. Each moment a challenge. There are simply not enough minutes in the day or days in the week to keep up.

For the parent of a child who is suffering, the first part of life to be lost is caring for themselves. Your child and family come first. You stop eating well. There is no time for exercise, much less activities to feed your soul. Meditation, reading, yoga, time with your husband, hiking all fall away to be filled with counselors, appointments, money, questions, fear, guilt. As the parent, you must be standing up to fight for the wellbeing of your child. Seeking self-care is a must during this time even though it may feel selfish and possibly like sticking your head in the sand.

Taking care of yourself can give you the strength to manage what comes. You may face judgement from family, friends, church groups, and school. Kids with depression, anxiety with or without cutting can miss significant amounts of school. Some societies accept this, most blame the parent for not getting the child there. There is lack of understanding and there can be consequences for the child and parents. A mother shared with me recently that she is being taken to court due to her daughter missing so much school. This judgment can also be seen from family friends. Friendships can be lost because of differing ideology on treatment, lack of support, blame, faith, or cultural divides. It is important to find a group who can be understanding and supportive of your parenting and choices. It is your choice how your child is treated through her mental health crisis. It is a journey as individual as a fingerprint that you can navigate with support and guidance.

Chapter 9:

You Can Do This

That first moment of finding gashes on the forearm of your child under their sleeve is a moment of anguish which is quickly followed by the feeling of inadequacy. How do I help my child when she feels so horrible that she would take a razor and cut her skin over and over? The way you help is to educate yourself and therefore empower yourself to help get what your daughter needs to stop cutting and be happy in life.

Jaqueline, a 15-year-old patient of mine came to me in crisis. Her mother walked into the clinic dragging

Jaqueline behind stating they had to be seen that day. The school had found cuts on her arm and she felt Jaqueline was suicidal. One of Jaqueline's friends saw her arm and told the school counselor. Even in a practice where there is a mental health side, the front staff tried to give her an appointment with one of the primary care providers. Of course, there were no openings. They came to me. This occurred right before lunch and I had finished up with my last patient a bit early. They entered the small room we use for mental health visits and we sat down together. It took ten minutes for Jacqueline's mom to calm down and start sharing. At first, she was talking in rapid succession about her own fears. Stating question after question without seeking an answer. How could this have happened? Why did she not tell me? How long has this been happening? Why did you do this? Where did you learn this? Was it at school? Do your friends do this? And so on. Jacqueline sat curled up in a ball in the chair, her head in her hands quietly crying. After some calming moments, mom was able to share Jaqueline's history. She is a successful student with very good grades. She is involved in multiple activities in school. She has lots of friends although mom has not seen them very much lately. Yes, she is not eating as well as she did. Mom attributes this to being so busy in school.

She goes to her room right after school most days and will take a nap. She will sometimes get up and join the family for dinner but sometimes will sleep straight through the night and have a very hard time getting up and going to school. She used to love doing her make-up and hair every morning. The last time it was done to Jaqueline's standards may have been two months ago.

Mom went to wait in another room and Jaqueline was given her time to talk about what was happening. She shared openly with intermittent tears that she had been cutting for months. It started when she was angry with her boyfriend. She used a razor and made short cuts all over her forearm in all directions. There had been conflict in her home and her grades had been slipping. She talked for over an hour and was breathing better. We discussed the highway and ways to get off. She came up with ideas herself for distraction techniques. Once mom came back in, we discussed the use of medicines, the pathophysiology of what was happening in her brain at this time, and how the medicine works including possible side effects. We discussed how journaling can help process emotions and that counseling is a very useful tool. Jaqueline, like some of my other patients, was not open to try seeing a counselor, not even with encouragement and a thorough description of how they work. So, she started seeing me twice weekly for a time. We worked on coping strategies and how she can gain control in her life. She started naming her emotions and the events around them. She was able to define moments or situations which were triggers for her. She then put a behavior plan in place for when one of those situations occurred, she would know what do differently to ensure a better outcome than what had occurred in the past.

Jacqueline did cut again while we were working together. This time on her left thigh. It was more like scratches than deep cuts. Later she had the urge but did not take action. That day, she came into my office and sat down as if she owned the place and said, "I had the urge and instead walked around my house singing my grandmother's favorite song in my head. I did not cut." She was empowered and smiling ear to ear. The urge may never go away, although I hope it will. But she now has the power and confidence to choose rather than a pathway out of her control determining her actions. She now sees me every other month and soon I expect our visits to become even less frequent. Once they are safe, I let them decide how often they need to come in based upon their comfort.

It is an honor when they say, I can make it on my own. See you later.

The process begins with the discovery of something happening with your child and deciding help is needed. The medical system today is not equipped to manage children who are having mental health crisis. Many may not view the circumstance as a crisis, but it absolutely is one. Pediatric offices all care and want to assist, but are constrained by time demands and for some, limited education in the field of mental health. There are so many providers with varied education, experience, and dedication. It is a must to know what the provider knows and how they treat. It is your choice who your child sees. The personality match between your child and the provider is imperative. If there is no connection, there will be no trust and no progress. Be aware of the system, its limitations, and how it is set up. In an emergency, you need to be in a place where they are capable of providing the care needed or can find it for you.

There are many reasons a child may cut. Cutting is not a standalone phenomenon. It is a symptom of underlying feelings and struggle. They need a diversion from the current state. Self-harm may be learned from others or discovered on their own by accident. The children hide their behavior out of lack of understanding, fear of judgement, fear of being in trouble, shame, trying to protect their parents or some think it is just not a big deal.

Cutting typically comes out of seeking control of pain or seeking to feel. These are based on emotional states. The child's brain is not like an adult's. They are born without understanding or definitions of emotions. They have to develop these over time. It is a slow process occurring over many years. Understanding where your child is in this process helps communication and enables you to teach along the way. The development of executive function occurs when the pre-frontal cortex completes development sometime in the twenties. Prior to that children do not have the skills to completely self-regulate emotions. Some never attain the skill.

The brain is complex and has trillions of connections. Cutting can be a symptom of anxiety, depression, ADHD or be secondary to another diagnosis. These conditions are mediated by the neurochemical structure of the brain. The symptoms are due to an imbalance of neurotransmitters in the synapses between cells. The behaviors are not a choice for your child, you as a parent did not cause them. The body is like a bathtub. Able to hold only so much of what life brings. A child has a smaller bathtub and does not have the skills to understand how to regulate what comes in and goes out. When stressed or overflowing, the brain reverts to the innate instinct for fight or flight where the body is primed physically to literally take out the threat or run for your life. Either way, with or without fighting or running, the nervous system has been activated. A child only knows they feel amped up, not why, and will act out behaviors accordingly. Once they begin reacting to a stimulus with a behavior, a pathway is created in the brain. The more that pathway is used, the larger and more solid it becomes like a highway. The steps between stimulus and result are often not in the child's control or even awareness.

Treatment is based upon the underlying cause. There are many tools available and all which apply should be used. The medications available are safe and very effective when used properly. The old adage that getting 50 percent better is a success is no longer valid. Our children deserve to heal 100 percent. For the tools including counseling and meditation to work, the brain needs to be in a place it can learn and grow. It needs to have neurotransmitters which are balanced and operating effectively to propagate signals, not diminished and creating symptoms. Many techniques are available such as 1:2 breathing, box breathing, focus on peripheral vision, meditation, CBT, EMDR, and so many more. It is hard to find the match and what works for your child, but it can be accomplished.

There are so many obstacles in your path but knowing they are there makes them manageable if not conquerable. Taking one step at a time, one after the other gets you to the destination. The destination will be determined by the needs of your unique child. It cannot be mandated by you, your doctor or the system. We must listen and adjust trajectory as needed. Be aware and open, then embrace your mama bear to take down whatever obstacle presents itself. You are not alone. There is no blame – only love.

End Notes

(1) Spiegel, Alix. "The History and Mentality of Self-Mutilation." NPR Morning edition. June 10, 2005.

(2) Lang, Susan S. "Self-injury is prevalent among college students, but few seek medical help, study by Cornell and Princeton researchers finds." *Cornell Chronicle.* June 5, 2006.

Seligson, Susan. "Cutting: The Self-Injury Puzzle." *BU Today.* April 4, 2013.

American Psychiatric Association. Diagnostic and statistical manual of mental disorders, 5th ed., (DSM-5). Washington, DC: American Psychiatric Publishing; 2013.

(3) Saarni C. Emotional Development in Childhood. In: Tremblay RE, Boivin M, Peters RDeV, eds. Lewis M, topic ed. *Encyclopedia on Early Childhood Development* [online]. http://www.child-encyclopedia.com/emotions/according-experts/emotional-development-childhood. Published September 2011. Accessed March 3, 2019.

(4) Morin, Amanda. "Social and Emotional Skills: What to expect at different ages." *Understood. WEB*

(5) Barkley, Russell A, PhD, ABPP. "Executive Functioning: Nature, Assessment, and Management." Continuing Ed Course. Net. November 14, 2018.

(6) Stahl, Stephen M. "Stahl's Essential Psychopharmacology". Cambridge University Press. Fourth Edition 2013.

(7) St. George, Donna. "How mindfulness practices are changing an inner-city school." *The Washington Post.* November 13, 2016.

Suggested Reading

I have found wonderful moments in each of these books. Please read what resonates with you. From each book, find ideas or guidance which is pertinent to your situation and your child. I do not feel one book has all the answers to a situation, but everything you read will further your knowledge base, giving you more of a foundation on which to stand.

Books:
Anxious by Jospeh LeDoux

First, We Make the Beast Beautiful by Sarah Wilson

The 7 Habits of Highly Effective Teens by Sean Covey

The Subtle Art of Not Giving a F*ck by Mark Manson

Make Your Bed by Admiral William H. McRaven

How to Talk So Kids Will Listen & Listen So Kids Will Talk by Adele Faber & Elaine Mazlish

Helping Teens Who Cut by Michael Hollander, PhD

Project Semicolon by Amy Bleuel

How to Teach Meditation to Children by David Fontana & Ingrid Slack

A Mindfulness-Based Stress Reduction Workbook for Anxiety by Bon Stahl, Phd, Florence Meleo-Meyer, MS, MA and Lynn Koerbel, MPH

Acknowledgments

Thank you to Angela Lauria and The Author Incubator's team, as well as to David Hancock and the Morgan James Publishing team for helping me bring this book to print.

Thank You

The journey to find this book and the journey that has now begun can seem as if you are at the bottom of a well. From that vantage point, you may not be able to see light at all or there may be just the lightest glow. Thank you for taking the time to read these words and to seek hope for your child. The process toward understanding and fighting for the health of your child is worthwhile and a must. Together, we can navigate the system. Each moment of education and clarity is a step up in that well. It's a stairway that enables you to climb out and have the tools to find and attain treatment for your child.

I invite you to reach out to me at www.underthesleeve. com to learn about a special four-week program in which we spend four two-hour sessions together going through each step of the process as it applies to your child and family. We will discuss each event in your child's life including development, school, and behaviors. We will discuss how these behaviors could be consistent with mental health diagnoses then what you have already tried to help relieve your child's suffering. What was beneficial for your child and what was not. I will go over with you the pathophysiology as it applies to your unique child and options for treatment. I will advise (not diagnose, this is not intended to take the place of a physician's care) on when to seek medical care and who might be the best fit for you and your family from the choices available to you. Then I will help you navigate the system to find the personality matches needed to assist your child in feeling safe and heard. Obstacles will be encountered which we will discuss. You will have support and direction every step of the way.

If your child is cutting, there is hope, and there is help. To connect with me, learn more about the ideas discussed in this book, and discover a practical program that can help your child please visit www.underthesleeve.com or text +1-503-828-0402 (normal message rates apply).

You may also listen to a free recorded message by calling +1-503-828-0402.

Your first introductory consultation is always free and there is no obligation. I encourage you to reach out today.

About the Author

Dr. Stacey Winters is a board-certified pediatrician who started her work with children over 20 years ago. She has fought the battle to attain appropriate pediatric mental health care as both a doctor and a mom. Her desire is to reach as many kids and families as possible to provide direction 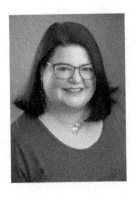 through education in the hopes to decrease pain and lend a hand for children with any type of mental illness to find success and happiness. She has treated hundreds of children and supported their families both in the clinic and hospital setting. Varied experiences, exposure, success, and struggles have given her a unique perspective and the ability to perceive beyond appearances.

She lives in Oregon with her beautiful daughter and the lovingly titled "animal herd." She loves reading, cooking, exploring, and learning.

Contact: DrStacey@underthesleeve.com

CPSIA information can be obtained
at www.ICGtesting.com
Printed in the USA
FSHW011651310720
72602FS